PREGNANCY JOURNEY

By

DR. JACOB WILLIAMS

CONTENTS

• **INTRODUCTION**

Each lady is unique. Their encounters of pregnancy are as well. Few out of every odd lady has similar side effects or even similar side effects starting with one pregnancy then onto the next.

Additionally, in light of the fact that the early side effects of pregnancy frequently imitate the side effects you could encounter just previously and during monthly cycle, you may not understand you're pregnant.

What follows is a portrayal of probably the most widely recognized early side effects of pregnancy. You ought to realize that these side effects might be brought about by different things other than being pregnant. So the way that you notice a portion of these side effects doesn't be guaranteed to mean you are pregnant. The best way to tell without a doubt is with a pregnancy test.

CHAPTER ONE

WAYS TO GET PREGNANT

You are prepared to get pregnant. Presently. When you are prepared to begin a family, holding up is the last thing you need to do.

In spite of the fact that The life-giving force of earth plays a part in the timing, there are a few things you can do - - or not do - - to assist with expanding your possibilities getting pregnant quickly. Peruse on for seven master endorsed ways to get pregnant.

1.Get a predisposition exam.

Before you formally begin attempting, get an exam. Get some information about pre-birth nutrients that have folic corrosive, which safeguards against some birth deserts, for example, spina bifida. Folic corrosive works during the beginning phases of pregnancy, so that is the reason it's essential to ensure you're getting enough folic corrosive even before you get pregnant.

"Do this the cycle before you begin attempting," says Paula Hillard, MD, a teacher of obstetrics and gynecology at Stanford College. "Assuming you have any basic clinical issues, they should be taken care of before you can securely become pregnant."

2. Get to know your cycle.

What amount do you are familiar your feminine cycle? Truly understanding assists you with knowing when you're generally fruitful, says Hillard. Ovulation is the best chance to get pregnant. "This is an ideal opportunity to zero in on engaging in sexual relations," Hillard says.It assists with becoming mindful of the indications of ovulation, like an adjustment of your cervical bodily fluid. It typically turns out to be slender and elusive when you are generally prolific. A few ladies may likewise feel an uneven twinge of torment.

Ovulation expectation units can likewise assist you with anticipating the best chance to get pregnant, says James Goldfarb, MD, overseer of the barrenness administration at the Cleveland Facility in Cleveland. Besides the fact that they help can guarantee you that you are ovulating, "assuming you are having rare intercourse, this lets you know whenever to have it to build your possibilities getting pregnant," he says.

This is the carefully guarded secret: The principal day of your feminine period is viewed as the very first moment. "Begin testing on day nine and continue onward until you get a positive," prompts Joanne Piscitelli, MD, an academic partner of gynecology at Duke College Clinical Center in Durham, N.C. Ladies with a 28-day cycle will generally ovulate on day 14. Yet, numerous ladies have longer or more limited cycles, so projecting a wide net can assist you with being certain.

Imagine a scenario where you've been utilizing conception prevention. Do you have to stand by some time prior to attempting to get pregnant? Not actually, says Goldfarb. "Quite a while back, the customary way of thinking was to stand by a specific measure of time subsequent to halting conception prevention to attempt to get pregnant yet that is presently false. You can begin attempting to consider just after you stop anti-conception medication," Goldfarb says. The main thing to remember is that you could get pregnant before you get your period, so following ovulation might be troublesome, and sorting out your due date may be more diligently. Thus, "certain individuals might feel better holding on until they get one period all alone," he says.

3. Try not to stress over the best situations for getting pregnant.

Legends flourish about the best situations for getting pregnant, yet they are only that - - fantasies. There is actually no logical proof saying that the minister position is superior to the lady being on top with regards to expanding your possibilities making a child.

"Once in a long while, a lady's cervix is in a surprising position where certain positions can have an effect," Goldfarb tells WebMD.

Certain gravity-resisting positions, like sitting or remaining during intercourse, nonetheless, may deter sperm from voyaging upstream. "It's a question of gravity [and] you don't believe all the semen should run out - - and semen are fast little critters," Hillard says.

4. Remain in bed just after intercourse.

You have presumably heard this one - - lie in bed with your feet in the air subsequent to having intercourse to build your possibilities getting pregnant. The decision? Not (thoroughly) valid.

"It's solid counsel to lay in bed for 10 to 15 minutes after intercourse, yet you needn't bother with your feet in the air," Goldfarb says. "Your pelvis doesn't move when you put your legs in the air." Don't go the restroom during this time it is possible that, he says. "Assuming you stand by 10 to 15 minutes, the sperm that will get into the cervix will be in the cervix."

5. Try not to go overboard.

Engaging in sexual relations consistently in any event, during ovulation won't be guaranteed to build your possibilities getting pregnant. "As a general rule, each and every night around the hour of ovulation helps increment your possibility getting pregnant," Goldfarb says. Sperm can satisfy 5 days inside your body. The best idea is to engage in sexual relations routinely - - while you're ovulating, and when you're not.

Discussing sperm, "wearing tight-fitting dress can adversely influence sperm count," Piscitelli says. So too can investing energy in hot tub or Jacuzzi. Your man's PDA propensities may likewise additionally have serious room for improvement. A concentrate in the diary Fruitfulness and Sterility showed that men who utilized a sans hands gadget with a PDA and kept their telephone near their gonads had more unfortunate sperm quality.

They could have to pass on the edamame and other soy food varieties for some time, as well. Men who eat a ton of soy food sources might have a lower sperm focus than men who don't eat soy food sources.

6. De-stress some way you can.
Do whatever it takes not to become worried about beginning a family. You might feign exacerbation assuming somebody says, "Simply unwind and it will work out," however stress can really impede ovulation. So the more loosened up you are, the better!

Whatever helps you de-stress is fine, for however long it's solid. "There is some proof that needle therapy can assist with diminishing pressure and increment your possibilities becoming pregnant," Goldfarb says. What's more, in spite of the fact that drinking an excess of liquor while attempting to get pregnant isn't shrewd, a glass of wine won't do any harm.

7. Carry on with a solid life.

Practicing is a solid propensity - - particularly in the event that it helps keep you at your optimal weight. Very much like anything more, however, you can get an overdose of something that is otherwise good. "An excessive amount of activity can cause you not to ovulate," Goldfarb says.

What's excessively? It very well might be different for various ladies. In the event that you are a bad-to-the-bone exerciser and are as yet getting your period routinely, your activity routine is probably not an issue, he says. In any case, Goldfarb adds, your feminine period isn't the main thing to go on the off chance that you are practicing too vigorously. "The principal thing that happens is that you have a more limited last part of your cycle. You ought to have a period 14 days after you ovulate, however a lot of activity can abbreviate this stage." This would be the principal hint that you want to reduce your wellness routine. He proposes following what amount of time it requires for you to get a period after you ovulate as the most effective way to be aware without a doubt.

Goldfarb says the most ideal way to build your possibilities getting pregnant while getting the medical advantages of normal activity is to do direct activity - - think energetic strolling - - over two hours every week (or if nothing else 30 minutes, 5 days per week).

Quit smoking to expand your possibilities getting pregnant," Hillard says. Beside the wide range of various negative wellbeing impacts of smoking, this terrible propensity additionally diminishes fruitfulness. "It influences estrogen levels and ovulation."

Furthermore, don't stress a lot over your day organizer. "85% of ladies will become pregnant in somewhere around one year of endeavoring,"

● **CHAPTER TWO**

● **INCEPTION OF PREGNANCY**

Another individual is made when the components of a powerful sperm converge with those of a fruitful ovum, or egg. Prior to this association both the spermatozoon (sperm) and the ovum have relocated for impressive distances to accomplish their association. Various effectively motile spermatozoa are saved in the vagina, go through the uterus, and attack the uterine (fallopian) tube, where they encompass the ovum. The ovum has shown up there after expulsion from its follicle, or container, in the ovary. After it enters the cylinder, the ovum loses its external layer of cells because of activity by substances in the spermatozoa and from the covering of the tubal wall. Loss of the external layer of the ovum permits various spermatozoa to infiltrate the egg's surface. Just a single spermatozoon, in any case, ordinarily turns into the treating organic entity. Whenever it has entered the substance of the ovum, the atomic top of this spermatozoon isolates from its tail. The tail progressively vanishes, however the head with its core makes due. As it goes toward the core of the ovum (at this stage called the female pronucleus), the head expands and turns into the male pronucleus. The two pronuclei meet in the focal point of the ovum, where their threadlike chromatin material arranges into chromosomes.

Initially the female core has 44 autosomes (chromosomes other than sex chromosomes) and two (X, X) sex chromosomes. Before preparation a sort of cell division called a decrease division gets the quantity of chromosomes the female pronucleus down to 23, including one X chromosome. The male gamete, or sex cell, additionally has 44 autosomes and two (X, Y) sex chromosomes. Because of a decreasing division happening before preparation, it, as well, has 23 chromosomes, including either a X or a Y sex chromosome at the time that it converges with the female pronucleus.

After the chromosomes consolidation and separation in a cycle named mitosis, the treated ovum, or zygote, as it is presently called, partitions into two equivalent estimated girl cells. The mitotic division gives every girl cell 44 autosomes, a big part of which are of maternal and a big part of fatherly beginning. Every girl cell likewise has either two X chromosomes, making the new individual a female, or a X and a Y chromosome, making it a male. The sex of the little girl still up in the air, hence, by the sex chromosome from the male parent.

Preparation happens in the uterine cylinder. How long the zygote stays in the cylinder is obscure, yet it likely arrives at the uterine depression around 72 hours after preparation. It is sustained during its section by the emissions from the mucous film coating the cylinder. When it arrives at the uterus, it has turned into a mulberry-like strong mass called a morula. A morula is made out of at least 60 cells. As the quantity of cells in a morula builds, the zygote shapes an empty bubblelike structure, the blastocyst. The blastocyst, sustained by the uterine emissions, drifts free in the uterine pit for a brief time frame and afterward is embedded in the uterine coating. Typically, the implantation of the blastocyst happens in the upper piece of the uterine covering.

➢ **Outline**

Pregnancy happens when a sperm prepares an egg after it's set free from the ovary during ovulation. The prepared egg then goes down into the uterus, where implantation happens. An effective implantation brings about pregnancy.

By and large, a full-term pregnancy endures 40 weeks. There are many elements that can influence a pregnancy. Ladies who get an early pregnancy conclusion and pre-birth care are bound to encounter a sound pregnancy and bring forth a solid child.

Knowing what's in store during the full pregnancy term is significant for observing both your wellbeing and the strength of the child. Assuming that you might want to forestall pregnancy, there are likewise powerful types of contraception you ought to remember.

CHAPTER THREE

SIDE EFFECTS OF PREGNANCY

You might see a few signs and side effects before you even take a pregnancy test. Others will seem weeks after the fact, as your chemical levels change.

I. Missed period

A missed period is one of the earliest side effects of pregnancy (and perhaps the most exemplary one). Notwithstanding, a missed period doesn't be guaranteed to mean you're pregnant, particularly in the event that your cycle will in general be sporadic.

There are numerous medical issue other than pregnancy that can cause a late or missed period.

II. Cerebral pain

Cerebral pains are normal in early pregnancy. They're generally brought about by changed chemical levels and expanded blood volume. Contact your PCP in the event that your migraines don't disappear or are particularly difficult.

III. **Spotting**

A few ladies might encounter light draining and spotting in early pregnancy. This draining is most frequently the aftereffect of implantation. Implantation normally happens one to about fourteen days after preparation.

Early pregnancy draining can likewise result from generally minor circumstances like a contamination or disturbance. The last option frequently influences the outer layer of the cervix (which is extremely delicate during pregnancy).

Draining can likewise here and there signal a serious pregnancy confusion, like premature delivery, ectopic pregnancy, or placenta previa. Continuously contact your primary care physician assuming you're concerned.

IV. **Weight gain**

You can hope to acquire somewhere in the range of 1 and 4 pounds in your initial not many long periods of pregnancy. Weight gain turns out to be more observable around the start of your subsequent trimester.

V. **Pregnancy-instigated hypertension**

Hypertension, or hypertension, now and again creates during pregnancy. Various elements can build your gamble, including:

i.   ☐being overweight or corpulent

ii.   ☐smoking

iii. ☐having an earlier history or a family background of pregnancy-initiated hypertension

iv. Acid reflux

Chemicals delivered during pregnancy can in some cases loosen up the valve between your stomach and throat. At the point when stomach corrosive holes out, this can bring about acid reflux.

VI. Stoppage

Chemical changes during early pregnancy can dial back your stomach related framework. Subsequently, you might become clogged up.

VII. Cramps

As the muscles in your uterus start to extend and grow, you might feel a pulling vibe that looks like feminine issues. On the off chance that spotting or draining happens close by your spasms, it could flag an unsuccessful labor or an ectopic pregnancy.

VIII. Back torment

Chemicals and weight on the muscles are the greatest reasons for back torment in early pregnancy. Later on, your expanded weight and moved focus of gravity might add to your back aggravation. Around half of all pregnant ladies report back torment during their pregnancy.

IX. **Pallor**

Pregnant ladies have an expanded gamble of pallor, which causes side effects like tipsiness and wooziness.

The condition can prompt untimely birth and low birth weight. Pre-birth care normally includes evaluating for weakness.

X. **Melancholy**

Somewhere in the range of 14 and 23 percent of all pregnant ladies foster melancholy during their pregnancy. The numerous natural and profound changes you experience can be contributing causes.

Make certain to let your primary care physician know if you don't feel like your typical self.

XI. A sleeping disorder

A sleeping disorder is one more typical side effect of early pregnancy. Stress, actual uneasiness, and hormonal changes can be contributing causes. A reasonable eating routine, great rest propensities, and yoga stretches can all assist you with getting a decent night's rest.

XII. Bosom changes

Bosom changes are quite possibly the earliest perceptible indication of pregnancy. Indeed, even before you're far enough along for a good test, your bosoms might start to feel delicate, enlarged, and by and large weighty or full. Your areolas may likewise expand and more delicate, and the areolae may obscure.

XIII. Skin inflammation

As a result of expanded androgen chemicals, numerous ladies experience skin break out in early pregnancy. These chemicals can make your skin oilier, which can obstruct pores. Pregnancy skin break out is typically transitory and clears up after the child is conceived.

XIV. **Regurgitating**

Regurgitating is a part of "morning disorder," a typical side effect that normally shows up inside the initial four months. Morning infection is many times the principal sign that you're pregnant. Expanded chemicals during early pregnancy are the primary driver.

XV. **Hip agony**

Hip agony is normal during pregnancy and will in general expansion in late pregnancy. It can have different causes, including:

☐ tension on your tendons

☐ sciatica

☐ changes in your stance

☐ a heavier uterus

XVI. **Loose bowels**

Loose bowels and other stomach related troubles happen habitually during pregnancy. Chemical changes, an alternate eating routine, and added pressure are potential clarifications. On the off chance that looseness of the bowels endures in excess of a couple of days, contact your PCP to ensure you don't become dried out.

XVII. Stress and pregnancy

While pregnancy is normally a blissful time, it can likewise be a wellspring of stress. Another child implies enormous changes to your body, your own connections, and, surprisingly, your funds. Go ahead and your PCP for help on the off chance that you start to feel overpowered.

> **The main concern**

In the event that you figure you might be pregnant, you shouldn't depend entirely on these signs and side effects for affirmation. Taking a home pregnancy test or seeing your PCP for lab testing can affirm a potential pregnancy. A considerable lot of these signs and side effects can likewise be brought about by other medical issue, like premenstrual condition (PMS). Look into the early side

effects of pregnancy —, for example, how before long
they'll show up after you miss your period.

CHAPTER FOUR

PREGNANCY STEP BY STEP

Pregnancy weeks are gathered into three trimesters, every one with clinical achievements for both you and the child.

I.   FIRST TRIMESTER

A child develops quickly during the principal trimester (weeks 1 to 12). The baby starts fostering their mind, spinal line, and organs. The child's heart will likewise start to thump.

During the principal trimester, the likelihood of an unsuccessful labor is somewhat high. As per the American School of Obstetricians and Gynecologists (ACOG), it's assessed that around 1 of every 10 pregnancies end in unnatural birth cycle, and that around 85% of these happen in the primary trimester.

Look for guaranteed help in the event that you experience the side effects of unsuccessful labor.

II. SECOND TRIMESTER

During the second trimester of pregnancy (weeks 13 to 27), your medical care supplier will probably play out a life structures check ultrasound.

This test really takes a look at the baby's body for any formative irregularities. The experimental outcomes can likewise uncover the sex of your child, assuming you wish to figure out before the child is conceived.
You'll presumably start to feel your child move, kick, and punch within your uterus.

Following 23 weeks, a child in utero is thought of "practical." This implies that it could endure living beyond your belly. Children conceived this early frequently have serious clinical issues. Your child has a greatly improved possibility of being conceived sound the more you can convey the pregnancy.

III. THIRD TRIMESTER

During the third trimester (weeks 28 to 40), your weight gain will speed up, and you might feel more drained. Your child can now detect light as well as open and shut their eyes. Their bones are likewise framed.

As work draws near, you might feel pelvic uneasiness, and your feet might enlarge. Constrictions that don't prompt work, known as Braxton-Hicks withdrawals, may begin to happen long before you convey.

➢ The reality

Each pregnancy is unique, yet advancements will in all likelihood happen inside this general time period. Figure out additional about the progressions you and your child will go through all through the trimesters and pursue our I'm Anticipating that pamphlet should get week-by-week pregnancy direction.

• CHAPTER FIVE

• PREGNANCY TESTS

Home pregnancy tests are extremely precise after the primary day of your missed period. In the event that you come by a positive outcome on a home pregnancy test, you ought to plan a meeting with your primary care physician immediately. A ultrasound will be utilized to affirm and date your pregnancy

.

Pregnancy is analyzed by estimating the body's degrees of human chorionic gonadotropin (hCG). Additionally alluded to as the pregnancy chemical, hCG is created upon implantation. In any case, it may not be distinguished until after you miss a period.

After you miss a period, hCG levels increment quickly. hCG is distinguished through either a pee or a blood test.

Pee tests might be given at a specialist's office, and they're equivalent to the tests you can take at home.

Blood tests can be acted in a research center. hCG blood tests are probably all around as precise as home pregnancy tests. The thing that matters is that blood tests might be requested when six days after ovulation.

The sooner you can affirm you're pregnant, the better. An early finding will permit you to care more for your child's wellbeing. Get more data on pregnancy tests, for example, ways to keep away from a "misleading negative" result.

PREGNANCY AND VAGINAL RELEASE

An expansion in vaginal release is one of the earliest indications of pregnancy. Your creation of release might increment as soon as one to about fourteen days after origination, before you've even missed a period.

As your pregnancy advances, you'll keep on delivering expanding measures of release. The release will likewise will generally become thicker and happen all the more as often as possible. It's generally heaviest toward the finish of your pregnancy.

During the last a long time of your pregnancy, your release might contain dashes of thick bodily fluid and blood. This is classified "the ridiculous show." It very well may be an early indication of work. You ought to inform your PCP as to whether you have any dying.

Typical vaginal release, or leukorrhea, is slender and either clear or smooth white. It's additionally gentle smelling.

On the off chance that your release is yellow, green, or dark with a solid, horrendous scent, it's viewed as strange. Unusual release can be an indication of a disease or an issue with your pregnancy, particularly on the off chance that there's redness, tingling, or vulvar enlarging.

On the off chance that you assume you have unusual vaginal release, let your medical services supplier know right away. Look into vaginal release during pregnancy.

PREGNANCY AND URINARY PLOT CONTAMINATIONS (UTIs)

Urinary plot contaminations (UTIs) are perhaps of the most well-known difficulty ladies experience during pregnancy. Microbes can get inside a lady's urethra, or urinary parcel, and can climb into the bladder. The embryo comes down on the bladder, which can make the microorganisms be caught, causing a contamination.

Side effects of a UTI typically incorporate torment and consuming or continuous pee. You may likewise insight:
☐ shady or blood-touched pee
☐ pelvic torment

☐lower back torment

☐fever

☐queasiness and retching

Almost 18% of pregnant ladies foster a UTI. You can assist with forestalling these contaminations by purging your bladder much of the time, particularly when sex. Drink a lot of water to remain hydrated. Try not to involve douches and brutal cleansers in the genital region. Contact your medical care supplier on the off chance that you have side effects of a UTI. Contaminations during pregnancy can be perilous on the grounds that they increment the gamble of untimely work.

When gotten early, most UTIs can be treated with anti-infection agents that are successful against microscopic organisms yet ok for use during pregnancy. Heed the guidance here to forestall UTIs before they even beginning.

CHAPTER SIX

FOOD VARIETIES AND DRINKS TO KEEP AWAY FROM DURING PREGNANCY

One of the primary things individuals realize when they're pregnant is what they can't eat. It very well may be a genuine bummer in the event that you're a major sushi, espresso, or uncommon steak fan.

Fortunately, there's more you can eat than what you can't. You simply need to figure out how to explore the waters (the low mercury waters, that is). You'll need to give close consideration to what you eat and drink to remain sound .

Certain food sources ought to just be eaten seldom, while others ought to be stayed away from totally. The following are 11 food sources and refreshments to stay away from or limit while pregnant.

I.   **High mercury fish**

Mercury is an exceptionally harmful component. It has no known safe degree of exposureTrusted Source and is most usually tracked down in dirtied water.

In higher sums, it tends to be poisonous to your sensory system, resistant framework, and kidneys. It might likewise create serious formative issues in kids, with antagonistic impacts even in lower sums.

Since it's found in contaminated oceans, huge marine fish can aggregate high measures of mercury. Consequently, it's ideal to keep away from high mercury fish while pregnant and breastfeeding.

High-mercury fish you need to stay away from include:
☐ shark

☐ swordfish

☐ lord mackerel

☐ fish (particularly bigeye fish)

☐ marlin

☐ tilefish from the Inlet of Mexico

☐ orange roughy

In any case, it's vital to take note of that not all fish are high in mercury — simply specific sorts.

Devouring low mercury fish during pregnancy is extremely solid, and these fish can be eaten up to multiple times per weekTrusted Source, as per the Food and Medication Organization (FDA).

Low mercury fish are ample and include:

☐ anchovies

☐ cod

☐ fumble

☐ haddock

☐ salmon

☐ tilapia

☐trout (freshwater)

Greasy fish like salmon and anchovies are particularly great choices, as they are high in omega-3 unsaturated fats, which are significant for your child.

II. Half-cooked or crude fish

This one will be intense for you sushi fans, yet entirely it's a significant one. Crude fish, particularly shellfish, can cause a few diseases. These can be viral, bacterial, or parasitic contaminations, for example, norovirus, Vibrio, Salmonella, and Listeria.

A portion of these contaminations may just influence you, causing lack of hydration and shortcoming. Different contaminations might be given to your child with serious, or even deadly, outcomes.

Pregnant ladies are particularly vulnerable to listeria diseases. As a matter of fact, as indicated by the Habitats for Infectious prevention and Counteraction (CDC), pregnant ladies depend on multiple times more likelyTrusted Source to get contaminated by Listeria than everyone. Pregnant Hispanic ladies are multiple times more in danger.

This microbes can be tracked down in soil and defiled water or plants. Crude fish can become contaminated during handling, including smoking or drying.

Listeria microorganisms can be passed to your child through the placenta, regardless of whether you're not giving any indications of disease. This can prompt unexpected labor, unnatural birth cycle, stillbirth, and other serious medical issues, as per the CDCTrusted Source.

It's certainly encouraged to keep away from crude fish and shellfish, including numerous sushi dishes. However, sit back and relax, you'll appreciate it substantially more after child is conceived and it's more secure to eat once more.

III. **Half-cooked, crud**

A portion of similar issues with crude fish influence half-cooked meat, as well. Eating half-cooked or crude meat builds your gamble of contamination from a few microorganisms or parasites, including Toxoplasma, E. coli, Listeria, and Salmonella.

Microorganisms might compromise the soundness of your little one, potentially prompting stillbirth or extreme neurological diseases, including scholarly incapacity, visual deficiency, and epilepsy.

While most microorganisms are found on the outer layer of entire bits of meat, different microbes might wait inside the muscle strands.

A few entire cuts of meat — like tenderloins, sirloins, or ribeye from hamburger, sheep and veal — might be protected to eat when not cooked the whole way through. Nonetheless, this possibly applies when the piece of meat is entire or whole, and totally cooked outwardly.

Cut meat, including meat patties, burgers, minced meat, pork, and poultry, ought to never be devoured crude or half-cooked. So keep those burgers on the barbecue great until further notice.

Franks, lunch meat, and store meat are likewise of concern, which is now and then amazing for pregnant individuals. These sorts of meat might become tainted with different microbes during handling or stockpiling. Pregnant ladies shouldn't consume handled meat items except if they've been warmed until steaming hot.

IV. Crude eggs

Crude eggs can be sullied with the Salmonella microorganisms.

Side effects of salmonella diseases incorporate fever, sickness, spewing, stomach spasms, and looseness of the bowels.

Nonetheless, in uncommon cases, the disease might cause cramps in the uterus, prompting untimely birth or stillbirth.

Food sources that normally contain crude eggs include:

☐ softly fried eggs

☐ poached eggs

☐ hollandaise sauce

☐ natively constructed mayonnaise

☐ some natively constructed salad dressings

☐ hand crafted frozen yogurt

☐ natively constructed cake icings

Most business items that contain crude eggs are made with purified eggs and are protected to consume. In any case, you ought to continuously peruse the mark to ensure.

To play it safe, make a point to constantly cook eggs completely or utilize purified eggs. Save those very runny yolks and custom made mayo until after child makes their presentation.

V. **Organ meat**

Organ meat is an incredible wellspring of various supplements.

These incorporate iron, vitamin B12, vitamin A, zinc, selenium, and copper — which are all really great for yourself and child. Nonetheless, eating an excess of creature based vitamin A (preformed vitamin A) isn't suggested during pregnancy.

Consuming an excess of preformed vitamin A, particularly in the principal trimester of pregnancy, can prompt intrinsic contortions and unsuccessful labor.

Albeit this is generally associatedTrusted Source with vitamin An enhancements, it's ideal to keep your utilization of organ meats like liver to only a couple of ounces one time each week.

VI. Caffeine

You might be one of the large numbers of people who love their everyday cups of espresso, tea, soda pops, or cocoa. You're most certainly not the only one with regards to our affection for caffeine.

Pregnant individuals are by and large encouraged to restrict their caffeine admission to under 200 milligrams (mg) each day, as per the American School of Obstetricians and Gynecologists (ACOG).

Caffeine is consumed rapidly and passes effectively into the placenta. Since children and their placentas don't have the fundamental compound expected to process caffeine, undeniable levels can develop.

High caffeine admission during pregnancy has been displayed to confine fetal development and increment the gamble of low birth weight at conveyance.

Low birth weight — characterized as under 5 lbs., 8 oz. (or on the other hand 2.5 kg) — is related with an expanded riskTrusted Wellspring of newborn child demise and a higher gamble of persistent sicknesses in adulthood.

So watch out for your everyday cup of joe or soft drink to ensure child doesn't have openness to a lot of caffeine.

VII. Crude fledglings

Your solid plate of mixed greens decision may not be liberated from rebel fixings, all things considered. Crude fledglings, including horse feed, clover, radish, and mung bean sprouts, might be polluted with Salmonella.

The sticky climate expected by seeds to begin growing is great for these sorts of microorganisms, and they're exceptionally difficult to wash off.

Therefore, you're encouraged to keep away from crude fledglings out and out. Notwithstanding, sprouts are protected to consume after they have been cooked, as indicated by the FDATrusted Source.

VIII. Unwashed produce

The outer layer of unwashed or unpeeled products of the soil might be sullied with a few microorganisms and parasites.

These incorporate Toxoplasma, E. coli, Salmonella, and Listeria, which can be procured from the dirt or through dealing with.

Tainting can happen whenever during creation, gather, handling, capacity, transportation, or retail. One perilous parasite that might wait on foods grown from the ground is called Toxoplasma.

Most of individuals who get toxoplasmosis have no side effects, while others might feel like they have seasonal influenza for a month or more.

Most babies who are tainted with the Toxoplasma microbes while still in the belly have no side effects upon entering the world. Be that as it may, side effects, for example, visual impairment or scholarly handicaps may developTrusted Source sometime down the road.

Furthermore, a little level of tainted infants have serious eye or mind harm upon entering the world.

While you're pregnant, it's vital to limit the gamble of contamination by completely washing with water, stripping, or cooking foods grown from the ground. Keep it up as a beneficial routine after child shows up, as well.

IX. Unpasteurized milk, cheddar, and organic product juice

Crude milk, unpasteurized cheddar, and delicate matured cheesesTrusted Source can contain a variety of destructive microorganisms, including Listeria, Salmonella, E. coli, and Campylobacter. (These are most likely sounding recognizable at this point.)

The equivalent goes for unpasteurized juice, which is likewise inclined to bacterial defilement. These diseases can all have dangerous consequencesTrusted Hotspot for an unborn child.

The microorganisms can be normally happening or brought about by defilement during assortment or capacity. Sanitization is the best method for eliminating any hurtful microscopic organisms, without changing the healthy benefit of the items.

To limit the gamble of diseases, eat just sanitized milk, cheddar, and organic product juice.

X. **Liquor**

It's encouraged to totally try not to drink liquor when pregnant, as it builds the gamble of unsuccessful labor and stillbirthTrusted Source. Indeed, even a modest quantity can adversely influence your child's cerebrum developmentTrusted Source.

Drinking liquor during pregnancy can likewise cause fetal liquor condition, which includes facial distortions, heart deformities and scholarly handicap.

Since no amount of alcoholTrusted Source has been shown to be protected during pregnancy, keeping away from it altogether is suggested.

XI. Handled unhealthy foods

There could be no more excellent time than pregnancy to begin eating supplement thick food varieties to help both you and your developing minimal one. You'll require expanded measures of numerous fundamental supplements, including protein, folate, choline, and iron.

Likewise a fantasy you're "eating for two." You can eat as you regularly do during the principal semester, then, at that point, increaseTrusted Source by around 350 calories each day in your subsequent trimester, and around 450 calories each day in your third trimester.

An ideal pregnancy eating plan ought to mostly comprise of entire food sources, with a lot of supplements to satisfy yours and child's necessities. Handled low quality food is by and large low in supplements and high in calories, sugar, and added fats.

While some weight gain is important during pregnancy, abundance weight gain has been connected to numerous complexities and illnesses. These incorporate an expanded gamble of gestational diabetesTrusted Source, as well as pregnancy or birth difficulties.

Stick to feasts and bites that emphasis on protein, vegetables and organic products, sound fats, and fiber-rich carbs like entire grains, beans, and bland vegetables. Simply relax, there are bunches of ways of slipping veggies into your feasts without forfeiting taste.

➢ **The primary concern**

At the point when you're pregnant, it's fundamental to keep away from food varieties and refreshments that might seriously jeopardize you and your child.

Albeit most food sources and drinks are entirely protected to appreciate, some, similar to crude fish, unpasteurized dairy, liquor, and high mercury fish, ought to be stayed away from.

Furthermore, a few food varieties and refreshments like espresso and food sources high in added sugar, ought to be restricted to advance a sound pregnancy.

To get familiar with what food varieties you ought to eat during pregnancy, look at this article: Good dieting During Pregnancy.

• FOOD SOURCES TO EAT WHEN YOU'RE PREGNANT

Pregnant? Over the top hungry? Searching for a bite that will satisfy your stomach and your child? You're most likely hearing it a great deal: Eating nutritious food sources while pregnant is fundamental.

We're here to make your storage room into an all inclusive resource of solid and scrumptious food sources that will give your child the best beginning to life.

While building your smart dieting plan, you'll need to zero in on entire food sources that give you higher measures of the great stuff you'd require when not pregnant, for example,

☐ protein

☐ nutrients and minerals

☐ sound sorts of fat

☐ complex carbs

☐ fiber and liquids

The following are 13 very nutritious food sources to eat when you're pregnant to assist with ensuring you're hitting those supplement objectives.

I.   Dairy items

During pregnancy, you really want to consume additional protein and calcium to address the issues of your developing minimal one. Dairy items like milk, cheddar, and yogurt ought to be on the agenda.

Dairy items contain two kinds of top notch protein: casein and whey. Dairy is the best dietary wellspring of calcium, and gives high measures of phosphorus, B nutrients, magnesium, and zinc.

Yogurt, particularly Greek yogurt, contains more calcium than most other dairy items and is particularly valuable. A few assortments likewise contain probiotic microbes, which support stomach related wellbeing.

Assuming you're lactose prejudiced, you may likewise have the option to endure yogurtTrusted Source, particularly probiotic yogurt. Check with your PCP to check whether you can test it out. An entire universe of yogurt smoothies, parfaits, and lassi could pause.

II. Vegetables

This gathering of food incorporates lentils, peas, beans, chickpeas, soybeans, and peanuts (also known as a wide range of breathtaking recipe fixings!).

Vegetables are extraordinary plant-based wellsprings of fiber, protein, iron, folate, and calcium — all of which your body needs a greater amount of during pregnancy. Folate is one of the most fundamental B nutrients (B9). It's vital for yourself and child, particularly during the primary trimester, and even previously.

You'll require no less than 600 micrograms (mcg) of folateTrusted Source each day, which can be a test to accomplish with food sources alone. Be that as it may, including vegetables can assist with getting you there alongside supplementation in light of your PCP's suggestion.

Vegetables are for the most part exceptionally high in fiber, as well. A few assortments are likewise high in iron, magnesium, and potassium. Consider adding vegetables to your eating regimen with dinners like hummus on entire grain toast, dark beans in a taco salad, or a lentil curry.

III. Yams

Yams are not just delightful cooked around 1,000 different ways, they're likewise wealthy in beta carotene, a plant compound that is changed over into vitamin An in your body.

Vitamin An is fundamental for child's turn of events. Simply look out for unreasonable measures of creature based wellsprings of vitamin A, for example, organ meats, which can cause toxicityTrusted Source in high sums.

Fortunately, yams are a more than adequate plant-based wellspring of beta carotene and fiber. Fiber keeps you full longer, lessens glucose spikes, and works on stomach related wellbeing (which can truly help assuming that pregnancy stoppage hits).

For a fab brekky, attempt yams as a base for your morning avocado toast.

IV. Salmon

Smoked on an entire wheat bagel, teriyaki barbecued, or slathered in pesto, salmon is a welcome expansion to this rundown. Salmon is wealthy in fundamental omega-3 unsaturated fats that have a large group of advantages.

These are tracked down in high sums in fish, and assist with building the mind and eyes of your child and could actually assist with expanding gestational length.

Be that as it may, stand by: Have you been told to restrict your fish consumption because of the mercury and different pollutants found in high mercury fish? You can in any case eat greasy fish like salmon.

Here are the high mercury fish to avoidTrusted Source:

☐ swordfish

☐ shark

☐ ruler mackerel

☐ marlin

☐ bigeye fish

☐ tilefish from the Bay of Mexico

In addition, salmon is a rare example of regular wellsprings of vitamin D, which is missing for the greater part of us. It's significant for bone wellbeing and safe capability.

V. Eggs

Those fantastic, consumable eggs are a definitive wellbeing food, as they contain a smidgen of pretty much every supplement you want. A huge egg contains around 80 calories, top notch protein, fat, and numerous nutrients and minerals.

Eggs are an extraordinary wellspring of choline, an imperative supplement during pregnancy. It's significant in child's mental health and forestalls formative irregularities of the mind and spine.

A solitary entire egg contains around 147 milligrams (mg)Trusted Wellspring of choline, which will draw you nearer to the ongoing suggested choline admission of 450 mg for every dayTrusted Source while pregnant (however more investigations are being finished to decide whether that is sufficient).

Here are the absolute best ways of cooking eggs. Attempt them in spinach feta wraps or a chickpea scramble.

VI. Broccoli and dull, mixed greens
Nothing unexpected here: Broccoli and dull, green vegetables, for example, kale and spinach, pack in so large numbers of the supplements you'll require. Regardless of whether you love eating them, they can frequently be squirreled into a wide range of dishes.

Benefits incorporate fiber, L-ascorbic acid, vitamin K, vitamin A, calcium, iron, folate, and potassium. They're a mother lode of green goodness.

Including servings of green veggies is a productive method for pressing in nutrients and fight off clogging because of all that fiber. Vegetables have likewise been connected to a decreased gamble of low birth weightTrusted Source.

Attempt this kale eggs Florentine recipe or mix a few spinach into a green smoothie and you won't actually know it's in there.

VII. Lean meat and proteins
Lean hamburger, pork, and chicken are incredible wellsprings of excellent protein. Hamburger and pork are likewise plentiful in iron, choline, and other B nutrients — all of which you'll require in higher sums during pregnancy.

Iron is a fundamental mineral that is involved by red platelets as a piece of hemoglobin. You'll require more iron since your blood volume is expanding. This is especially significant during your third trimester.

Low degrees of iron during ahead of schedule and mid-pregnancy might cause lack of iron frailty, which expands the gamble of low birth weightTrusted Source and different confusions.

It tends to be difficult to cover your iron necessities with feasts alone, particularly assuming that you foster a repugnance for meat or are veggie lover or vegetarian. In any case, for the people who can, eating lean red meat consistently may assist with expanding how much iron you're getting from food.

Master tip: Matching food varieties that are plentiful in L-ascorbic acid, for example, oranges or ringer peppers, alongside iron-rich food varieties may likewise assist with expanding assimilation.

Prepare some L-ascorbic acid rich tomato cuts on that turkey burger or prepare this steak and mango salad.

VIII. Berries
Berries hold a ton of goodness in their minuscule bundles like water, solid carbs, L-ascorbic acid, fiber, and cell reinforcements.

Berries have a generally low glycemic record esteem, so they shouldn't cause significant spikes in glucose.

Berries are likewise an extraordinary bite, as they contain both water and fiber. They give a great deal of flavor and sustenance, however with somewhat couple of calories.

Probably the best berries to eat while pregnant are blueberries, raspberries, goji berries, strawberries, and acai berries. Look at this blueberry smoothie for some motivation.

IX. Entire grains

Not at all like their refined partners, entire grains are loaded with fiber, nutrients, and plant compounds. Think oats, quinoa, earthy colored rice, wheat berries, and grain rather than white bread, pasta, and white rice.

A few entire grains, similar to oats and quinoa, likewise contain a considerable lot of protein. They likewise hit a couple of buttons that are in many cases ailing in pregnant individuals: B nutrients, fiber, and magnesium. There are such countless approaches to adds entire grains to any dinner, yet we're particularly preferring this quinoa and simmered yam bowl.

X. Avocados

Avocados are a strange organic product since they contain a ton of monounsaturated unsaturated fats. This makes them taste rich and rich — ideal for adding profundity and smoothness to a dish.

They're additionally high in fiber, B nutrients (particularly folate), vitamin K, potassium, copper, vitamin E, and L-ascorbic acid.

As a result of their high satisfied of sound fats, folate, and potassium, avocados are an incredible decision during pregnancy (and consistently).

The solid fats assist with building the skin, cerebrum, and tissues of your little one, and folate might assist with forestalling brain tube surrenders, formative anomalies of the mind and spine, for example, spina bifida.

Potassium might assist with easing leg squeezes, a symptom of pregnancy for certain ladies. Avocados contain more potassiumTrusted Source than bananas, as a matter of fact.

Attempt them as guacamole, in servings of mixed greens, in smoothies, and on entire wheat toast, yet in addition as a substitute for mayo or harsh cream.

XI. Dried organic product

Dried organic product is by and large high in calories, fiber, and different nutrients and minerals. One piece of dried natural product contains similar measure of supplements as new natural product, just without all the water and in a lot more modest structure.

One serving of dried natural product can give an enormous level of the suggested admission of numerous nutrients and minerals, including folate, iron, and potassium.

Prunes are plentiful in fiber, potassium, and vitamin K. They're normal diuretics and might be exceptionally useful in alleviating stoppage. Dates are high in fiber, potassium, iron, and plant compounds.

Be that as it may, dried organic product additionally contains high measures of normal sugar. Make a point to stay away from the sweetened assortments, which contain significantly more sugar.

Albeit dried organic product might assist with expanding calorie and supplement consumption, consuming more than each serving in turn is for the most part not suggested.

Take a stab at adding a little part to a path blend in with nuts and seeds for an in a hurry protein-and fiber-filled nibble.

XII. Fish liver oil

Fish liver oil is produced using the sleek liver of fish, most frequently cod. It's wealthy in the omega-3 unsaturated fats EPA and DHA, which are fundamental for fetal cerebrum and eye advancement.

Enhancing with fish oil might help safeguard against preterm conveyance and may help fetal eye improvement. Fish liver oil is likewise extremely high in vitamin D, of which many individuals don't get enough. It could be profoundly advantageous for the people who don't consistently eat fish or supplement with omega-3 or vitamin D.

A solitary serving (1 tablespoon or 15 milliliters) of fish liver oil gives more than the suggested day to day admission of omega-3, vitamin D, and vitamin A.

Be that as it may, it's not prescribed to consume more than one serving each day, as an excess of preformed vitamin A can be perilous for your child. Elevated degrees of omega-3 may likewise have blood-diminishing impacts.

Low mercury fish like salmon, sardines, canned light fish, or pollock can likewise assist with getting you to your omega-3 objectives.

XIII. Water

Let's assume it with me: We as a whole need to remain hydrated. What's more, pregnant people particularly. During pregnancy, blood volume increments by around 45 percentTrusted Source.

Your body will channel hydration to your child, however in the event that you don't watch your water consumption, you might become dried out yourself.

Side effects of gentle lack of hydration incorporate migraines, tension, sluggishness, terrible mind-set, and diminished memory.

Expanding your water admission may likewise assist with easing clogging and decrease your gamble of urinary parcel diseases, which are normal during pregnancy.

Common rules suggest that pregnant ladies drink around 80 ounces (2.3 liters) of water day to day. Be that as it may, the sum you truly need fluctuates. Check with your primary care physician for a proposal in light of your particular requirements.

Remember that you additionally get water from different food sources and drinks, like organic product, vegetables, espresso, and tea.

Master tip: Have a go at keeping a reusable water bottle close by so you can extinguish your thirst over the course of the day.

• CHAPTER SEVEN

• CONCLUSION

Your developing child is simply holding back to gulp up that large number of supplement thick food varieties from a balanced eating plan of entire grains, products of the soil, lean proteins, and solid fats.

There's an entire universe of scrumptious choices that give you and your child all that you'll require. Keep your medical care group educated regarding your eating decisions and let them guide you on an arrangement with any essential enhancements.